WATER WORKS:

Unleashing Of Kidney-Friendly Flavored Water For A Refreshing And Healthful Hydration

Ashley R. Whitlow

TABLE OF CONTENT

INTRODUCTION

Everyone is aware of the health benefits of water.

An adult and a kid will have a different percentage of water in their bodies. Every day, our bodies lose 2500 ml of water via excretion, perspiration, and other processes. About 900 ml of fluids are obtained from our meals, 350 ml are produced by our bodies, and the remaining portion should be consumed (between 1 and 1.5 liters).

What Makes Drinking Water So Crucial?
For instance, water handle the movement of nutrients and waste out of your body. In addition to ensuring that nutrients are digested for intestinal absorption, it also controls your body's temperature, which is crucial in the current heat wave.

Why is water intake crucial for your kidneys?
Water are necessary for your kidneys to operate

properly. You can produce enough urine to transport waste materials when you are well-hydrated. You may have observed that when you are thirsty, the color of your pee darkens.

This is due to the fact that it has increased in concentration. Additionally, you need to drink enough water for your blood to easily circulate to your kidneys and other organs. On its own, severe dehydration may harm the kidneys.

If you have end-stage renal disease and are receiving dialysis, this changes.
Water consumption has to be drastically reduced for dialysis patients since they cannot excrete enough water.

A condition known as hyponatremia, or too little sodium in the blood, may be brought on by excessive water consumption. Low sodium levels will enable more water to enter the cells, causing them to expand, since sodium regulates the body's fluid balance.

Hyponatremia may also happen in individuals who have renal failure, are taking diuretics, are professional athletes who are drinking and perspiring, or who are exercising in very hot conditions. You should thus carefully balance your fluid requirements if you have renal illness to prevent throwing off the ratio of your essential minerals.

Is water the only healthy drink available?
The best approach to hydrate is with plain water. However, most of us don't wish to always consume just water. Additionally, hot water is unpleasant, and at certain seasons of the year, there is nothing better than a hot beverage. Fortunately, there are healthier alternatives to water. Water may also be modified. As long as you choose a brand that doesn't include extra sodium or potassium, sparkling water is acceptable. You should watch out for certain nutrients. Steer clear of sugary drinks. Additionally, watch how much potassium you ingest.

Hyperkalemia, which happens when you have too much potassium in your blood because your kidneys cannot get rid of the extra potassium, is a risk for people with renal disease, especially late stages. You must constantly ingest potassium for your body to operate normally, but you must exercise care to avoid having too much potassium in your system.

Flavored water For hydration and cooling throughout the summer, infused water has gained popularity. You may put your preferred fruit and herbs in a pitcher of water, then let it alone for a few hours. The fruit or herb taste will be more prominent the longer you leave it standing.

It's crucial to choose components with less potassium. Blackberries, blueberries, cherries, cranberries, cucumber, raspberries, strawberries, and citrus fruits are all healthy options (oranges, however, should be avoided since they contain higher potassium). You can muddle it. On a hot

day, flavored water is quite appealing to many individuals.

The facts The proper hydration intake is crucial for those with renal illness. This often entails increasing your fluid intake if you have early-stage kidney disease, but you will likely be told to significantly reduce your fluid intake if you have end-stage renal failure or are receiving dialysis. While simple water is the healthiest beverage for your kidneys, other liquids including coffee, green tea, low-potassium juices, and flavored water are all entirely appropriate.
Coconut water and sugary, fizzy drinks should be avoided.

So what beverages need to be avoided?
People with renal issues should take extra caution to steer clear of a few drinks. To name a few: Coconut water. The majority of individuals can drink coconut water, which is often promoted as a healthy substitute for sports drinks. It has been demonstrated to increase

urine potassium even in healthy individuals, therefore it should only be used in moderation.

Coconut water or coconut milk should not be consumed if you have been told to lower your potassium intake. sodas, including diet sodas. Chronic renal disease risk has been linked to the daily use of two or more fizzy beverages. There is a lot of phosphorus in cola and other beverages. Due to its high sugar content, soda should be used in moderation or not at all. Diet Coke is not healthier for you since it has been shown to increase the risk of end-stage renal disease and artificial sweeteners may have a negative impact on your insulin levels.
Prunes juice. Prunes have a high potassium content as well.

CHAPTER 1: FLAVORED WATER

1. Pineapple-Mint Flavored Water

Serving per recipe:5

Serving size: 1 cup

For this recipe, you will need

1/2 cup fresh pineapple

6 fresh mint leaves

5 cups water

How To Prepare

Chop mint leaves, chop the pineapple.

Add all ingredients to a pitcher, Pour in 5 cups of water, and refrigerate for 4-8 hours or overnight. Pour into a cup and serve.

2. Watermelon-Rosemary Flavored Water

Serving per recipe: 5

Serving size: 1 cup

For this recipe, you will need

1 cup of diced watermelon

5 small stems of fresh rosemary

5 cups of water

How to prepare

Rinse and rosemary stem, and add all ingredients to a pitcher. Pour in 5 cups of water and refrigerate for 4-8 hours or overnight. Pour into a cup and serve.

3. Cucumber-Lemon Flavored Water

Serving per recipe: 5

Serving size: 1 cup

For This Recipe, You Will Need

1/2 medium cucumber

1/2 lemon

5 fresh basil leaves, 5 fresh mint leaves

5 cups water

How To Prepare

Finely chop basil and mint leaves. slice the cucumber and lemon.

Add all ingredients to a jar, Pour in 5 cups of water, and refrigerate for 4-8 hours or overnight. Pour into a cup and serve.

4. Citrus Water Flavored water

Serving per recipe: 5

Serving size: 1 cup

For This Recipe, You Will Need

5 cups of water

1/2 orange, 1/2 lemon, 1/2 lime

How to prepare

Slice the citrus into thin rounds, and put in a bowl. Using the end of a wooden spoon, press it until just a little juice comes out, but be careful not to completely pulverize them. into a jar and add 5 cups of water. Let sit for 3-4 hours in the refrigerator and then enjoy.

5. Lemon Berry Water Flavored water

Serving per recipe: 5

Serving size: 1 cup

For This Recipe, You Will Need

1 lemon, cut into 5

1 cup of raspberries or strawberries

5 cups of water

How to prepare

In a bowl, mash the berries with a fork or wooden spoon a little (don't make it a paste). Transfer into a jar, and add in the slices of the lemon. Add 5 cups of water. Refrigerate for 4-6 hours or overnight. Pour into a cup and serve.

6. Cinnamon Apple Water Flavored water

Serving per recipe: 5

Serving size: 1 cup

For This Recipe, You Will Need

5 small sticks of cinnamon

2 apples

5 cups of water

How to prepare

Slice the apple.

In a jar add the sliced apples and cinnamon, Pour in 5 cups of water and refrigerate for 4-8 hours or overnight. Pour into a cup and serve.

7. Pineapple-Ginger Mint Flavored Water

Serving per recipe: 5

Serving size: 1 cup

For This Recipe, You Will Need

2 cups of chopped pineapple

1 fresh ginger root

5 sprigs of mint

5 cups of water

How to prepare

Peel the ginger and slice it tiny.

In a jar add pineapple chunks, sliced ginger, and mint sprigs. Pour in 5 cups of water and refrigerate for 4-8 hours or overnight. Pour into a cup and serve.

8. Blackberry_Sage Flavored Water

Serving per recipe: 5

Serving size: 1 cup

For This Recipe, You Will Need

1 cup fresh blackberries

2 sage leaves

5 cups water

How To Prepare

Rinse and mashed the blackberries.

Add the berries and sage leaves in pitcher Pour in 5 cups of water and refrigerate for 4-8 hours or overnight. Pour into a cup and serve.

9. Mint_Lemon Flavored Water

Raspberry-lime water

Serving per recipe: 5

Serving size: 1 cup

For this recipe, you will need

5 cups water

1 lemon

5 mint sprigs

1/4 cup fresh raspberries

How To Prepare

1 Thinly slice lime.

12 Finely chop mint leaves.

Add all ingredients to a pitcher.

Refrigerator for 4-8 hours or overnight. Pour into a cup and serve.

10. Grape -Lemon-Mint Flavored Water

Serving per recipe: 5

Serving size: 1 cup

For this recipe, you will need

5 cups of water

1/3 lemon

1 cup of grapes

5 mint sprigs

How to prepare

Rinse the grape, mint sprigs, and lemon.

Cut the grape into two halves, and slice the lemon. Put in a jar pour 5 cups of water and refrigerate for 4-8 hours or overnight. Pour into a cup and serve.

11. Raspberry Apple Flavored Water

Serving per recipe: 5

Serving size: 1 cup

For this recipe, you will need

1/2 cup of raspberries

1 big apple

5 cups of water

How to prepare

Wash your berries and fruit

Cut your raspberries into 2 halves

Slice your apple into small size
Pour in 5 cups of water and refrigerate for 4-8 hours or overnight. Pour into a cup and serve.

12. Berry Apple Flavored Water

Serving per recipe: 5
Serving size: 1 cup
For this recipe, you will need
1 apple
1/2 cup of berries
5 cups of water

How to prepare

Wash your berries and your apple, cut the berries into 2 halves, slice your apple, put in a jar, pour in 5 cups of water, and refrigerate for 4-8 hours or overnight. Pour into a cup and serve.

13. Mint Apple flavored Water

Serving per recipe: 5
Serving size: 1 cup
For this recipe, you will need
5 cups of water

5 mint sprigs
2 apple

How to prepare
Rinse the apple and the mint leaves
Slice the apple, pour the sliced apples and mint leaves into a jar, pour in 5 cups of water and refrigerate for 4-8 hours or overnight. Pour into a cup and serve.

14. Grape And Mint Flavored Water
Serving per recipe: 5
Serving size: 1 cup
For this recipe, you will need
5 cups of water
5 mint sprigs
1 cup of grapes

How to prepare
Rinse the grape and the mint leaves
Slice the grape into 2 halves, pour the sliced grapes and mint leaves into a jar, pour in 5 cups of water, and refrigerate for 4-8 hours or overnight. Pour into a cup and serve.

15. Strawberry And Grape Flavored Water

Serving per recipe: 5

Serving size: 1 cup

For this recipe, you will need

5 cups of water

1/2 cup of strawberries

10 grapes

How to prepare

Rinse the grape and cut them into 2 halves, pour in the diced strawberry and grapes into a jar, add 5 cups of water, and refrigerate for 4-8 hours or overnight. Pour into a cup and serve.

16. Black Grape Pineapple Flavored Water

Serving per recipe: 5

Serving size: 1 cup

For this recipe, you will need

5 cups of water

1/2 cup of grapes

10 cube-size pineapple

How to prepare

Rinse and cut the grape into 2 halves, pour in the pineapple and grapes into a jar, add 5 cups of water, and refrigerate for 4-8 hours or overnight. Pour into a cup and serve.

17. Strawberry And Mint Flavored Water

Serving per recipe: 5
Serving size: 1 cup
For this recipe, you will need
5 cups of water
1 cup of cube-cut strawberries
5 mint sprigs

How to prepare

Rinse the mint sprigs.

Pour the cut strawberry into 2 halves. in a jar put in the strawberry and mint sprigs, add 5 cups of water, and refrigerate for 4-8 hours or overnight. Pour into a cup and serve.

18. Cranberry- Mint-Flavored Water

Serving per recipe: 5
Serving size: 1 cup
For This Recipe, You Will Need

5 cups of water

1 cup of cranberry

5 mint sprigs

How to prepare

Rinse the cranberry and mint leaves

Put in a jar add water and refrigerate for 4-8 hours or overnight. Pour into a cup and serve.

19. Cranberry-Rosemary Flavored Water

Serving per recipe: 5

Serving size: 1 cup

For This Recipe, You Will Need

5 cups of water

1 cup of cranberry

5 small stems of fresh rosemary leaves

How to prepare

Rinse the rosemary the stem, cut the cranberry into halves, and rinse and transfer into a jar, Pour in 5 cups of water and refrigerate for 4-8 hours or overnight. Pour into a cup and serve.

20. Cranberry -Apple Flavored Water

Serving per recipe: 5
Serving size: 1 cup
For This Recipe, You Will Need
5 cups of water
1/2 cup of cranberry
1 Apple

How to prepare

Rinse the cranberry and cut it into 2 halves
Rinse the apple and slice
Put all ingredients in a jar pour in 5 cups of water and refrigerate for 4-8 hours or overnight. Pour into a cup and serve.

21. Blueberry- Peach-Mint Flavored Water

Serving per recipe: 5
Serving size: 1 cup
For This Recipe, You Will Need
5 cups of water
I cup of blueberries
1 peach

How to prepare

Rinse and slice the peach.

Rinse the blackberries

Combine all ingredients in a pitcher pour in 5 cups of water and refrigerate for 4-8 hours or overnight. Pour into a cup and serve.

22. Peach-Strawberry-Mint Flavored Water

Serving per recipe: 5

Serving size: 1 cup

For This Recipe, You Will Need

5 cups of water

1/2 cup of strawberries

1 peach

5 mint sprigs

How to prepare

Rinse the ingredients

Slice the peach

Combine all ingredients in a jar pour in 5 cups of water and refrigerate for 4-8 hours or overnight. Pour into a cup and serve.

23. Peach-Rosemary Flavored Water

Serving per recipe: 5

Serving size: 1 cup

For This Recipe, You Will Need
5 cups of water
5 small stems of fresh rosemary leave
2 peaches

How to prepare
Rinse all the ingredients.
Slice the peach
Put ingredients in a pitcher pour in 5 cups of water and refrigerate for 4-8 hours or overnight. Pour into a cup and serve.

24. Apple-Basil-Clementine Flavored Water
Serving per recipe: 5
Serving size: 1 cup
For This Recipe, You Will Need
5 cups of water
1/2 apple
5 basil leaves
1 clementine

How to prepare
Slice the apple, peel the clementine.

Put ingredients in a jar, pour in 5 cups of water, and refrigerate for 4-8 hours or overnight. Pour into a cup and serve.

25. Clementine-Blackberries-Clove flavored water

Serving per recipe: 5
Serving size: 1 cup
For This Recipe, You Will Need
5 cups of water
5 clementine
10 cloves
1 cup Blackberries

How to prepare
Crush the blackberries with the back of spoon in a small bowl. Add the cloves to the small saucepan after adding the liquid from the crushed blackberries. One of the clementines should be thinly sliced and added to the pan. Juice from the remaining clementine, which has been cut in half, is spread over everything before water is added.

For five to ten minutes, simmer the mixture over low heat. Carefully ladle the mixture into cups before serving. You may also combine all the prepared ingredients in a small teapot, add two cups of boiling water, and let it steep for five to ten minutes. The greatest time to enjoy this infusion is during the winter when clementines are in season and at their peak.

26. Lime-Cherry-Flavored Water

Serving per recipe: 5

Serving size: 1 cup

For This Recipe, You Will Need

5 cups of water

1-1/2 cup of cherry

1/2 lime

How to prepare

Slice the lime

Rinse the berries

Add ingredients to a pitcher, pour in 5 cups of water, and refrigerate for 4-8 hours or overnight. Pour into a cup and serve.

27. Cherry -Lemon-Mint Flavored Water

Serving per recipe: 5

Serving size: 1 cup

For This Recipe, You Will Need

5 cups of water

10 cherries

5 mint sprigs

3 slices of lemon

How to prepare

All the ingredients should be combined in a bowl, mashed together with a fork to release juice, then transferred to a jar and add water. Give the combination 10 to 15 minutes to settle so that the juice and water may combine. It may be left out on the counter or put in the refrigerator to cool.

NOTE

Measurements

Oz	Cup	Millimeters	Tablespoon	Teaspoon
8	1	238	16	48
6	3/4	177	12	36
5	2/3	158	11	32
4	1/2	118	8	24
3	1/3	79	5	16
2	1/4	59	4	12
1	1/8	30	2	6
0.5	1/16	15	1	3